ELIZABETH V. CARRINGTON

FERTILITY DIET RECIPES FOR NEWLY MARRIED

Yummy and Delicious Paths to Parenthood Through Simple Diets

ELIZABETH V. CARRINGTON

THANKS FOR PURCHASING MY BOOK!

Thank you immensely for choosing my "Fertility Diet Recipes for Newly Married" cookbook! In appreciation, I've crafted a special perk just for you. If you encounter any challenges or have questions about a recipe – whether it's adjusting ingredients or ensuring a perfect result – feel free to reach out. Your satisfaction is my top priority. Simply send an email to elizabethcarringtoncooks@gmail.com, detailing your query, and I'll promptly provide the solution you're seeking. Consider this my way of expressing gratitude and offering support on your fertility dietary journey.

Don't hesitate to take advantage of this offer. Your culinary success in the realm of fertility matters, and I'm here to assist you.

HAPPY COOKING!

TABLE OF CONTENTS

Chapter 1. Introduction

Nutrition has a vital role in fertility, regulating both male and female reproductive health. As a seasoned dietitian, I realize the tremendous influence that dietary choices may have on the delicate balance essential for healthy conception. In a day when lifestyle variables greatly impact general well-being, recognizing the role of diet in fertility is crucial.

Importance of Nutrition for Fertility

Nutrition forms the cornerstone of reproductive health, regulating hormone balance, egg and sperm quality, and general reproductive function. Essential nutrients including folic acid, zinc, omega-3 fatty acids, and antioxidants are important for sustaining reproductive health. A well-balanced diet not only encourages the formation of healthy eggs and sperm but also offers an ideal environment for implantation and fetal growth.

Moreover, keeping a healthy weight with good eating is vital for fertility. Both underweight and overweight disorders may negatively impair fertility by disturbing hormonal balance. For women, irregular menstrual periods and ovulatory dysfunction may come from insufficient or excessive body fat. In males, obesity has been associated with poorer sperm quality and testosterone levels. Thus, acquiring and maintaining a healthy weight is a major part of fertility optimization via diet.

COMMON CONCERNS OF NEWLY MARRIED COUPLES:

Newly married couples typically battle with similar worries surrounding fertility. Women may worry about irregular menstruation periods, while males could be worried about sperm quality and quantity. Nutritional choices may considerably alleviate these difficulties. Educating couples on the influence of food on reproductive health is vital in relieving anxiety.

Addressing lifestyle variables such as stress, poor sleep, and sedentary behaviors is vital. Nutrition, being an intrinsic aspect of lifestyle, may positively affect these parameters. Assuring couples that adopting a fertility-friendly diet may be a proactive move towards boosting their chances of conception can give them a feeling of empowerment and control over their fertility journey.

PURPOSE OF THE BOOK - "FERTILITY DIET RECIPES FOR NEWLY MARRIED":

The objective of this book is to serve as a thorough guide for newly married couples wishing to boost their fertility via diet. It combines my knowledge as a nutritionist with practical, tasty recipes geared to assist reproductive health. Readers should anticipate a comprehensive approach that goes beyond just nutritional instructions, incorporating lifestyle variables that contribute to fertility.

WHAT READERS CAN EXPECT:

A collection of expertly produced dishes meant to combine fertility-boosting ingredients. These meals will not only be nutritional but also tasty, making the road towards a fertility-friendly diet fun.

Recognizing that fertility is impacted by different lifestyle variables, the book will give practical guidance on stress management, appropriate sleep, and physical exercise. A holistic strategy is necessary for overall fertility optimization.

Structured meal plans will aid readers in organizing their weekly diet, ensuring they satisfy their nutritional requirements. In conclusion, this book aspires to be a trusted guide for couples commencing their reproductive journey. By combining evidence-based dietary counsel with delightful meals, it hopes to make the route to motherhood not only scientifically sound but also joyful. Through this resource, I strive to educate couples with the information and skills they need to make great food and lifestyle choices, establishing a firm foundation for a healthy and satisfying reproductive journey.

Chapter 2. Understanding Fertility Basics

The complexity of the reproductive system is a wonder of nature, as various variables harmonize to permit the production of life.

The reproductive system requires a complex balance between the male and female components. In men, the testes create sperm, whereas females contain ovaries that release eggs. Fertilization happens when sperm meets egg, resulting in the development of a zygote. This zygote undergoes cellular division, ultimately turning into an embryo and finally a fetus.

Crucial to this process is the menstrual cycle in females, controlled by hormonal variations. The pituitary gland releases follicle-stimulating

hormone (FSH) and luteinizing hormone (LH),
prompting the ovaries to create estrogen and
progesterone. These hormones control the
menstrual cycle, preparing the uterine lining for
a prospective pregnancy.

FACTORS INFLUENCING FERTILITY

1. *Hormonal Balance:* Hormones are the
conductors of this complicated symphony. Any
interruption in the delicate hormonal balance
might impair fertility. Conditions like polycystic
ovarian syndrome (PCOS) or irregular menstrual
periods may emerge from hormonal
abnormalities, impacting the ability to procreate.

2. *Nutrition and Fertility:* As a dietitian, I highlight
the role of nutrition in improving reproductive
health. Adequate consumption of important
nutrients, such as folate, zinc, and omega-3

fatty acids, enhances both male and female fertility. A well-balanced diet guarantees that the body has the required building blocks for reproductive activities.

3. *Lifestyle Choices:* Lifestyle variables greatly impact fertility. Smoking, heavy alcohol intake, and drug addiction may affect reproductive function. Maintaining a healthy weight is vital, since both underweight and overweight disorders may alter hormonal balance and menstrual regularity.

4. *Stress Management*: Chronic stress may severely affect fertility by disturbing hormonal balance. Incorporating stress-reduction strategies like mindfulness, yoga, or meditation may lead to a more suitable environment for conception.

Common Misconceptions concerning Fertility

1. Myth: Fertility is entirely a female problem.

Reality: Both couples contribute to fertility. Male variables, including sperm quality and quantity, are equally significant.

2. Myth: Conception is assured during ovulation.

Reality: While ovulation is the most fertile phase, it doesn't ensure conception. Various elements, including sperm health and uterine environment, play essential roles.

3. Myth: Age doesn't affect male fertility.

Reality: Advanced paternal age may impair sperm quality and raise the chance of genetic problems in kids.

4. Myth: A healthy lifestyle doesn't affect fertility.

Reality: Nutrition, exercise, and general lifestyle choices dramatically affect reproductive health for both men and women.

Understanding fertility includes grasping the complicated systems of the reproductive system and identifying the various elements impacting conception. As a dietician, I advocate for a holistic approach, stressing the crucial role of nutrition and lifestyle in promoting healthy fertility. By debunking prevalent myths, people may make educated decisions to increase their reproductive well-being.

Chapter 3: Nutritional Foundations for Fertility

Optimal fertility is a multidimensional element impacted by different circumstances, and one's nutrition stands as a crucial foundation. In this thorough guide, I will go into the fundamental nutrients required for reproductive health, detail foods rich in vitamins, minerals, and antioxidants that aid fertility, and underline the overarching value of a balanced diet in promoting general well-being.

Essential Nutrients for Reproductive Health

1. *Folate:* Known for its function in preventing neural tube abnormalities during pregnancy, folate is equally vital for both men and women in the preconception period. It assists in DNA synthesis and repair, playing a critical function in cell division. Leafy greens, beans, and fortified cereals are great sources.

2. *Omega-3 Fatty Acids*: These necessary fats are crucial for sperm production and motility. Fatty fish like salmon, chia seeds, and walnuts are rich in omega-3 fatty acids, leading to enhanced reproductive results.

3. *Vitamin D:* Beyond its function in bone health, vitamin D has been connected to reproductive success. Sun exposure, fatty fish, and fortified dairy products may help maintain healthy vitamin D levels.

4. *Iron:* Essential for oxygen delivery, iron is important for both male and female fertility. Incorporate lean meats, legumes, and leafy greens to guarantee an appropriate consumption.

5. *Zinc:* This mineral is crucial for sperm production and motility. Foods like oysters, lean meats, and seeds are great sources of zinc.

6. *Antioxidants:* Protecting cells from oxidative stress, antioxidants are crucial for reproductive health. Vitamins C and E, present in citrus fruits, berries, and nuts, play a critical role in neutralizing free radicals.

7. *Calcium:* Apart from its role in bone health, calcium is needed for smooth muscle action, including the uterus. Dairy products, fortified plant-based milk, and leafy greens are important calcium sources.

8. Protein: Adequate protein consumption is needed for the generation of reproductive hormones. Incorporate lean meats, poultry, eggs, and plant-based protein sources for a balanced approach.

FOODS RICH IN REPRODUCTIVE HEALTH-BOOSTING NUTRIENTS

1. Leafy Greens: Spinach, kale, and broccoli give an abundance of folate, iron, and other important elements required for reproductive health.

2. Berries: Packed with antioxidants, berries like blueberries and strawberries aid in general reproductive well-being.

3. Fatty Fish: Salmon, mackerel, and trout are good sources of omega-3 fatty acids, promoting sperm health and egg quality.

4. *Nuts and Seeds*: Almonds, walnuts, and chia seeds give a combination of healthy fats, protein, and antioxidants good for fertility.

5. *Colorful Vegetables*: Bell peppers, carrots, and sweet potatoes are rich in vitamins and minerals, boosting reproductive health.

6. *Lean Proteins:* Incorporate chicken, lean meats, tofu, and lentils to satisfy protein needs for hormone synthesis.

7. *Dairy or Fortified Plant-Based Alternatives:* These give key nutrients including calcium and vitamin D necessary for reproductive health.

8. *Whole Grains*: Quinoa, brown rice, and oats deliver complex carbs and fiber, boosting general well-being.

THE ROLE OF A BALANCED DIET IN FERTILITY

A balanced diet isn't only about individual nutrients; it's about establishing a harmonious nutritional environment that fosters general well-being. Excessive consumption of processed meals, sugary drinks, and trans fats might severely impair fertility. Opting for a vast and colorful assortment of whole meals offers a broad range of nutrients required for reproductive health.

Moreover, keeping a healthy weight is crucial for fertility. Both underweight and overweight situations may disturb hormonal balance, reducing menstruation regularity and sperm production. A balanced diet, along with regular physical exercise, supports a healthy weight and leads to enhanced reproductive results.

Improving fertility with diet takes a comprehensive approach. By ingesting a range of nutrient-dense meals, people may optimize their reproductive health and increase the probability of successful pregnancy. My purpose is to equip you with the information and resources to make informed nutritional choices, establishing a foundation for a healthy and satisfying reproductive journey.

Chapter 4. Fertility-Boosting Meals Throughout the Day

Breakfast for Fertility

01: Blueberry Muffins

Servings: 12 muffins| Prep Time: 15 minutes| Cooking Time: 20-25 minutes

Total Time: 35 minutes.

Nutritional Information (per serving):

Calories: 240 -Total Fat: 9g | Saturated Fat: 5g| Trans Fat: 0g | Cholesterol: 50mg| Sodium: 220mg| Total Carbohydrates: 36g | Dietary Fiber: 1g| Sugars: 18g| Protein: 4g

Ingredients:

- ❖ 2 cups all-purpose flour

- ❖ 1 cup granulated sugar
- ❖ 1 tablespoon baking powder
- ❖ 1/2 teaspoon salt
- ❖ 1/2 cup unsalted butter, melted
- ❖ 2 big eggs and 1 cup of milk
- ❖ 1 teaspoon vanilla extract
- ❖ 1 ½ cups fresh or frozen blueberries

INSTRUCTIONS:

1. Preheat the oven to 375°F (190°C). Line a muffin tray with paper liners or oil each cup.

2. In a large mixing basin, whisk together the flour, sugar, baking powder, and salt.

3. In a separate dish, whisk the eggs and then add the melted butter, milk, and vanilla extract. Mix thoroughly.

4. Pour the wet ingredients into the dry

ingredients and whisk until just incorporated. Be cautious not to overmix; the batter should be lumpy.

5. Gently incorporate in the blueberries, ensuring they are uniformly distributed throughout the batter.

6. Spoon the batter into the prepared muffin cups, filling each approximately two-thirds full.

7. Bake in the preheated oven for 20-25 minutes or until a toothpick inserted into the middle of a muffin comes out clean.

8. Allow the muffins to cool in the tray for 5 minutes before transferring them to a wire rack to cool fully

02: QUICHE

Serves:6 slices| Prep Time: 20 minutes|

Cooking Time: 45 to 60 minutes

Per Serving Nutritional Information:

320 calories| 20g of total fat| 9g of saturated fat| Trans Fat: 0g| 190 mg of cholesterol| 680 mg of sodium| 19g of total carbohydrates| One gram of dietary fiber| 2g of sugars| 16g of protein

Ingredients

- ❖ One pie crust (homemade or from the store)
- ❖ 1/2 cup chopped onion
- ❖ 1/2 cup diced bell pepper (any color)
- ❖ 1 cup diced cooked bacon or ham
- ❖ 1 cup shredded Swiss or Gruyère cheese
- ❖ Four big eggs
- ❖ One cup of milk

- ❖ 1/4 teaspoon grated nutmeg (optional)
- ❖ 1/2 teaspoon salt
- ❖ 1/4 teaspoon black pepper

INSTRUCTIONS:

1. Turn the oven on to 375°F, or 190°C. Transfer the pie crust to a 9-inch pie plate and reserve.

2. Cooked bacon or chopped ham should be softly browned in a pan. Take off the heat and put aside.

3. Saute the chopped onion and bell pepper in the same pan until they become tender. Take off the heat and put aside.

4. Combine the eggs, milk, nutmeg (if using), salt, and pepper in a mixing dish.

5. Arrange the sautéed veggies, grated cheese,

and ham or bacon in layers inside the pie shell.

6. Using a spoon, evenly distribute the egg mixture over the pie crust components.

7. Bake for 40 to 45 minutes, or until the top is golden brown and the middle is set, in a preheated oven.

8. Before slicing, let the quiche cool for ten minutes.

3. FRUIT SALAD FOR FERTILITY

Servings: 4 | Prep Time: 15 minutes

PER SERVING NUTRITIONAL INFORMATION:

120 calories | - 1g of total fat | - Saturated Fat: 0 g | - Trans Fat: 0g | There is no cholesterol | 5 milligrams of sodium | 30g of total carbohydrates | 6g of dietary fiber | 18g of

sugars | 2g of protein

INGREDIENTS:

- ❖ One cup of blueberries
- ❖ Two cups of fresh strawberries, hulled and cut in half.
- ❖ One cup of chunky pineapple

- ❖ One cup of peeled and sliced Kiwi
- ❖ 1 cup arils from pomegranates
- ❖ One tablespoon honey (to be drizzled over)
- ❖ One tablespoon of optional chia seeds

INSTRUCTIONS:

1. Combine the strawberries, blueberries, kiwi slices, pineapple pieces, and pomegranate arils in a large mixing dish.

2. Gently toss the fruits until well combined.

3. If preferred, drizzle some honey over the fruit salad to offer some sweetness and extra nutritious value.

4. For an additional dose of fiber and omega-3 fatty acids, you may optionally top the salad with chia seeds.

5. Toss the salad one more to make sure the chia seeds and honey are evenly coated.

6. For a cool and refreshing experience, serve the fertile fruit salad right away or store it in the refrigerator.

4. BANANA OAT MUFFINS

Servings: 12 muffins| Prep Time: 15 minutes|

Cooking Time: 20-25 minutes

NUTRITIONAL DATA FOR EACH MUFFIN:

120 calories| 1.5g of total fat| 0.5g of saturated fat| Trans Fat: 0g| 15 mg of cholesterol| 90 mg of sodium| 25g of total carbohydrates| 3g of dietary fiber| 10g of sugars| 3g of protein

INGREDIENTS:

- ❖ Two mashed, ripe bananas
- ❖ One big egg
- ❖ 1/4 cup honey or maple syrup
- ❖ 1/2 cup unsweetened applesauce
- ❖ 1 teaspoon vanilla essence
- ❖ One cup of traditional oats
- ❖ One cup of whole wheat flour;
- ❖ One teaspoon of powdered sugar
- ❖ Half a teaspoon of baking soda

- ❖ One-half teaspoon of cinnamon

- ❖ 1/2 cup milk (vegan or dairy)

- ❖ 1/4 teaspoon salt

- ❖ 1/4 cup chocolate chips (optional)

- ❖ Chopped nuts (optional)

INSTRUCTIONS

1. Set the oven's temperature to 350°F (175°C). Grease each cup or use paper liners to line a muffin pan.

2. Put the mashed bananas, applesauce, egg, vanilla extract, and honey (or maple syrup) in a big basin. Blend until well blended.

3. Combine the oats, whole wheat flour, baking soda, baking powder, cinnamon, and salt in another basin.

4. Stirring until just blended, gradually add the

dry ingredients to the wet components.

5. Add the milk and stir the mixture until it has a smooth texture. Add chocolate chips or chopped nuts, if preferred.

6. Using a spoon, scoop out the batter and fill each muffin cup to approximately two-thirds of the way.

7. Bake for 20 to 25 minutes, or until a toothpick inserted into the middle of a muffin comes out clean, in a preheated oven.

8. After the muffins have cooled in the pan for five minutes, move them to a wire rack to finish cooling.

5. Citrus Sticky Rolls

Servings: 12 rolls| Prep Time: 25 minutes| Cooking Time: 25-30 minutes

Nutritional data for each roll:

320 calories| 12g of total fat| 7g of saturated fat| Trans Fat: 0g| 30 mg of cholesterol| 180 mg of sodium| 48g of total carbohydrates| One gram of dietary fiber| Sugar content: 23g| 4g of protein

Ingredients: Dough Ingredients:

- ❖ 1/4 cup granulated sugar
- ❖ 1/4 cup melted unsalted butter
- ❖ 1 teaspoon salt
- ❖ 2 1/4 teaspoons active dry yeast
- ❖ 1 cup warm milk
- ❖ 3 1/2 cups of flour (all-purpose)

FOR THE FILLING:

- ❖ 1/2 cup softened unsalted butter
- ❖ 1/2 cup packed brown sugar
- ❖ One orange's zest
- ❖ One lemon's zest

FOR THE GLAZE OF CITRUS:

- ❖ Two teaspoons of fresh orange juice
- ❖ One cup of powdered sugar
- ❖ A tsp of freshly squeezed lemon juice
- ❖ One orange's zest (for garnish)

GUIDELINES:

FOR THE DOUGH

1. Dissolve the yeast in the warm milk in a small basin. Until foamy, let it rest for five minutes.

2. Combine the yeast mixture, sugar, flour, melted butter, and salt in a large mixing basin. Stir to produce a soft dough.

3. Place the dough on a floured board and knead it for five to seven minutes, or until it is elastic and smooth. After the dough has doubled in size, put it in a bowl that has been oiled, cover it with a moist towel, and let it rise in a warm location for an hour.

4. To make the filling, combine the melted butter, brown sugar, orange zest, and lemon zest in a small basin and stir until well-mixed.

PUT TOGETHER THE ROLLS:

5. Turn the oven on to 375°F, or 190°C. On a surface dusted with flour, roll out the dough into a rectangle.

6. Evenly distribute the citrus filling throughout the dough.

7. Forming a log, firmly roll the dough from the long side. Divide into 12 equal rolls.

8. After putting the rolls in a baking dish that has been buttered, give them another half hour to rise.

9. Bake the rolls for 25 to 30 minutes, or until they are golden brown, in a preheated oven.

FOR THE GLAZE OF CITRUS:

10. Combine the powdered sugar, orange juice, and lemon juice in a small basin and whisk until smooth.

11. Add some orange zest as a garnish and drizzle the heated rolls with the citrus glaze.

12. Warm up the citrus sticky rolls and savor them!

6. Avocado and Egg Toast

Servings: 2 servings | Prep Time: 10 minutes |
Cooking Time: 5 minutes

Nutritional data (per serving):

300 calories | 18g of total fat | 3g of saturated
fat | Trans Fat: 0g | 185 mg of cholesterol | 280
mg of sodium | 25g of total carbohydrates | 8g
of dietary fiber | 2g of sugars | 12g of protein

Ingredients:

- ❖ One ripe avocado
- ❖ Two slices of whole-grain bread
- ❖ Two sizable eggs
- ❖ To taste, add salt and pepper
- ❖ Optional red pepper flakes for more
  spiciness

❖ Chopped fresh parsley or chives (for garnish)

INSTRUCTIONS:

1. Toast the whole-grain bread pieces until they have the desired crispness.

2. Cut the ripe avocado in half, take out the pit, and scoop out the flesh into a dish while the bread is browning. Using a fork, mash the avocado and add salt and pepper to taste.

3. Fry the eggs in a nonstick pan until desired doneness. Aim for a runny yolk for a traditional avocado and egg toast.

4. Evenly distribute the mashed avocado over the pieces of toasted bread.

5. Gently top each toast with a fried egg that has been coated with avocado.

6. Add more salt and pepper to taste and season the eggs. Garnish the eggs with red pepper flakes if you're a spicy person.

7. Add some chopped parsley or fresh chives to the avocado and egg toast as a garnish.

8. Serve right away for a tasty and wholesome brunch or breakfast.

7. Sweet Oatmeal

Servings: 2 servings| Five minutes for preparation| Ten minutes for cooking

Nutritional data (per serving):

300 calories| - 6g of total fat| 3g of saturated fat| Trans Fat: 0g| 15 mg of cholesterol.| 80 mg of sodium| 52g of total carbohydrates| 5g

of dietary fiber | 18g of sugars

INGREDIENTS:

- ❖ 2 cups milk (vegan or dairy)
- ❖ 1 cup rolled oats
- ❖ Two teaspoons of maple syrup or honey
- ❖ 1/4 teaspoon cinnamon
- ❖ A pinch of salt
- ❖ half teaspoon vanilla extract
- ❖ Optional fresh fruit, nut, or seed topping

GUIDELINES:

1. Place rolled oats, milk, honey (or maple syrup), cinnamon, vanilla

essence, and a little amount of salt in a saucepan.

2. Over medium heat, bring the mixture to a mild boil, stirring from time to time.

3. Lower the heat to a simmer for 7 to 10 minutes, or until the mixture has thickened to your desired consistency and the oats are soft.

4. To give the oatmeal more time to thicken, take the skillet off the burner and leave it there for a few minutes.

5. Spoon the sugary oatmeal into a pair of dishes.

6. For more texture and taste, sprinkle fresh fruits, nuts, or seeds over top.

7. Present the sugary oatmeal warm and enjoy a nourishing and cozy morning meal.

8. BREAKFAST BURRITO

Servings: 2 burritos | Prep Time: 10 minutes | Cooking Time: 10 minutes | Total Time: 20 minutes

Nutritional details (per burrito):

450 calories | 24g of total fat | 8g of saturated fat | Trans Fat: 0g | 380 mg of cholesterol | 720 mg of sodium | 39g of total carbohydrates | 8g of dietary fiber | 5g of sugars | 23g of protein

Ingredients:

- ❖ 1/4 cup milk
- ❖ 4 big eggs
- ❖ 1/2 cup chopped bell peppers (any color)
- ❖ 1 tablespoon olive oil - salt and pepper to taste
- ❖ Half a cup of chopped onions
- ❖ 1/2 cup of tomatoes, diced
- ❖ 1/2 cup of black beans, cooked and seasoned

- ❖ 1/2 cup of shredded cheese (you may use Monterey Jack or cheddar, for example).

- ❖ Two sizable flour or whole wheat tortillas

- ❖ As a garnish, salsa, avocado, or sour cream (optional)

GUIDELINES:

1. Combine the eggs, milk, pepper, and salt in a bowl.

2. In a pan over medium heat, warm the olive oil. Cook the chopped onions and bell peppers until they become tender.

3. Cover the veggies in the pan with the egg mixture. Cook, stirring occasionally, until the eggs are well-cooked and scrambled.

4. Toss in cooked black beans and chopped

tomatoes with the eggs. Toss to blend thoroughly.

5. Top the egg mixture with the shredded cheese and allow it to melt.

6. Reheat the tortillas in a different pan or microwave, per the directions on the box.

7. Divide the egg and veggie mixture in half and place one-half on each tortilla.

8. To construct a burrito, fold the tortilla in half and wrap it up.

9. You may choose to add sour cream, avocado, or salsa as a garnish.

10. Present the warm breakfast burritos and enjoy your filling and delectable meal!

9. Yogurt Parfait

Servings: 2 servings| Prep Time: 10 minutes| Cooking Time:0 minutes| Total Time: 10 minutes

Nutritional data (per serving):

400 calories| - 15g of total fat| 2g of saturated fat| - Trans Fat: 0g| 10 mg of cholesterol| 80 mg of sodium| 50g of total carbohydrates| 7g of dietary fiber| 27g of sugars| 20g of protein

Ingredients:

- ❖ Two cups of plain or flavored Greek yogurt
- ❖ One cup of mixed berries (strawberries, blueberries, and raspberries)
- ❖ One cup of granola
- ❖ Two teaspoons of maple syrup or honey

❖ 1/4 cup of nuts or seeds, such as chia
   seeds or almonds

❖ Fresh mint leaves (as a garnish-optional)

INSTRUCTIONS:

1. Place 1/2 cup of Greek yogurt in the bottom
of each of two serving glasses or bowls.

2. Top each glass of yogurt with a layer of 1/4
cup granola.

3. The next layer should include a large handful
of mixed berries (strawberries, blueberries,
and raspberries).

4. Top each glass of fruit with a spoonful of
honey or maple syrup.

5. Repeat the layering process with an additional
1/2 cup Greek yogurt, 1/4 cup granola, and
more mixed berries.

6. For extra texture, sprinkle your preferred

nuts or seeds (almonds, chia seeds, etc.) over top of each parfait.

7. If preferred, garnish with fresh mint leaves.

8. Present the yogurt parfait right away as a wholesome and revitalizing morning or snack.

10. Fertility Omelet

Servings: 2 servings| Prep Time: 10 minutes| Cooking Time: 10 minutes

Total Time: 20 minutes

Nutritional Information (per serving):

Calories: 220| Total Fat: 16g| Saturated Fat: 5g| Trans Fat: 0g| Cholesterol: 390mg| Sodium: 320mg|-Total Carbohydrates: 4g Dietary Fiber: 1g| Sugars: 2g| Protein: 16g

INGREDIENTS:

- ❖ 4 big eggs
- ❖ 1 tablespoon olive oil
- ❖ 1/2 cup spinach, chopped
- ❖ 1/4 cup red bell pepper, diced
- ❖ 1/4 cup tomatoes, diced
- ❖ 1/4 cup feta cheese, crumbled
- ❖ 1/2 teaspoon dried oregano
- ❖ Salt and pepper (to taste)
- ❖ Fresh herbs for garnish (optional)

INSTRUCTIONS:

1. In a bowl, wash, beat and season the eggs with salt and pepper.

2. Over medium heat, heat olive oil in a non-stick skillet.

3. Add chopped spinach, red bell pepper, and

tomatoes to the skillet. Sauté until the veggies are somewhat softened.

4. Pour the beaten eggs over the veggies in the skillet.

5. Allow the eggs to set for a minute, then carefully raise the edges with a spatula, allowing the raw eggs to run below.

6. Sprinkle crumbled feta cheese and dried oregano equally over one side of the omelet.

7. Once the eggs are largely done but still somewhat runny on top, delicately fold the omelet in half using the spatula.

8. Cook for a further 1-2 minutes or until the eggs are thoroughly cooked and the cheese has melted.

9. Slide the fertile omelet onto a dish and garnish with fresh herbs if preferred.

10. Serve the omelet warm and enjoy a nutrient
-packed breakfast

Lunch for Fertility

01. Greek Wrap

Serves: 4| Prep Time: 15 minutes| Cooking Time: 10 minutes| Total Time: 25 minutes

Nutritional data (per serving):

450 calories| 30g of protein | 35g of carbohydrates| 20g of fat| 6g of fiber

Ingredients:

- ❖ Four whole wheat wraps
- ❖ A one-pound grilled and sliced chicken breast
- ❖ 1 cup halved cherry tomatoes
- ❖ 1 thinly sliced cucumber
- ❖ 1/2 thinly sliced red onion
- ❖ 1 cup crumbled feta cheese

- ❖ 1/4 cup of sliced Kalamata olives
- ❖ One-fourth cup of Greek dressing
- ❖ Recently harvested lettuce leaves

INSTRUCTIONS:

1. Cook the chicken on the grill until it's done, then cut it into strips.

2. Arrange every whole wheat wrapper and top with a couple of lettuce leaves.

3. Top each wrap with some grilled chicken, Kalamata olives, cucumber slices, cherry tomatoes, and feta cheese.

4. Cover each wrap's components with a drizzle of Greek dressing.

5. Tightly roll up the wrap after folding its sides inward toward the center.

6. Present right away and enjoy your Greek wrap!

02. Egg Salad Sandwich

Serves: 2| Prep Time: 10 minutes| Cooking Time: 10 minutes| Total Time: 20 minutes

INFORMATION ABOUT NUTRITION (PER SERVING):

400 calories| 20 g of protein| 25 g of carbs| 25 g of fat| Fiber: 5 grams

INGREDIENTS

- ❖ 6 hard-boiled eggs, peeled and diced
- ❖ 1/4 cup mayonnaise
- ❖ 1 tablespoon Dijon mustard
- ❖ 1/4 cup finely chopped celery
- ❖ 2 teaspoons finely chopped red onion.
- ❖ Four pieces of whole grain bread

❖ Salt and pepper to taste

❖ Slices of tomato (optional)

❖ Lettuce leaves

INSTRUCTIONS:

1. Put chopped hard-boiled eggs, mayonnaise, Dijon mustard, red onion, celery, and salt and pepper in a bowl. Stir well.

2. If preferred, toast the pieces of whole-grain bread.

3. Evenly distribute the egg salad between the two pieces of bread.

4. Top the egg salad with tomato slices and lettuce leaves, if preferred.

5. Place the remaining bread pieces on top to assemble sandwiches.

6. If desired, cut sandwiches in half before

serving.

03. Salmon Pinwheels

Serves: 4| Prep Time: 15 minutes| Cooking Time: 12 minutes| Total Time: 27 minutes

Nutritional Data (Per Serving):

350 calories| 25g of protein| 20g of carbohydrates| 18g of fat| 3g of fiber

Ingredients:

- ❖ Four 6-ounce salmon fillets
- ❖ 1/4 cup softened cream cheese
- ❖ Two teaspoons of chopped dill
- ❖ One tablespoon of juiced lemon
- ❖ Four big spinach tortillas

❖   Salt and pepper to taste

❖   One cup of young leaves of spinach

INSTRUCTIONS:

First, preheat the oven to 375°F, or 190°C.

2. After adding salt and pepper to the salmon fillets, bake them for 10 to 12 minutes in a preheated oven, or until they are cooked through.

3. Combine softened cream cheese, lemon juice, and chopped dill in a bowl.

4. Using a fork, break up the cooked salmon into little pieces.

5. Arrange the spinach tortillas and equally coat each one with the cream cheese mixture.

6. Arrange the salmon flake on top of the cream cheese layer and sprinkle baby spinach leaves on top.

7. Tightly roll each tortilla into a log, and then cut each log into pinwheels.

8. Present the pinwheels of salmon right away.

04. STEAK SANDWICH

Serves: 2| Prep Time: 15 minutes| Cooking Time: 10 minutes| Total Time: 25 minutes

NUTRITIONAL DATA (PER SERVING):

600 calories| 40g of protein| 40g of carbohydrates| 32g of fat| 4g of fiber

INGREDIENTS:

- ❖ 1 pound of sirloin steak
- ❖ 2 tablespoons of olive oil
- ❖ Thinly sliced onion
- ❖ sliced bell pepper

❖ Four pieces of your preferred bread; baguette or ciabatta work great.

❖ 1/4 cup of mayo

❖ 2 tsp Dijon mustard

❖ Fresh leaf lettuce

❖ Optional: slices of provolone or Swiss cheese

INSTRUCTIONS;

1. Sprinkle salt and pepper on the sirloin steak.

2. Add olive oil to a skillet and heat it to medium -high. Grill the steak for 3-4 minutes on each side, or until the desired doneness is achieved. Before slicing, let it a few minutes to rest.

3. Add more oil to the same pan if necessary, and sauté the bell pepper and onion slices until they are tender and caramelized.

4. Until they become golden brown, toast the bread pieces.

5. Combine mayonnaise and Dijon mustard in a small bowl.

6. Spread each bread slice's mayonnaise and Dijon mixture on one side.

7. Place sliced steak on half of the bread pieces, then add lettuce leaves and sautéed onion and bell pepper on top. Add pieces of cheese if desired.

8. Top with the remaining pieces of bread to finish the sandwiches.

9. Present the sandwich made with steak right away.

05. Fertility Protein Bowl

Serves: 2| Prep Time: 15 minutes| Cooking Time: 20 minutes| Total Time: 35 minutes

Nutritional Data (Per Serving):

600 calories| 25g of protein| 70g of carbohydrates| 28g of fat| 15g of fiber

Ingredients:

- ❖ 1 cup washed quinoa, 2 cups of water,1 tablespoon olive oil, and 1 cup of broccoli florets.
- ❖ One cup chopped sweet potato
- ❖ One cup chopped kale
- ❖ One cup of cooked and drained black beans
- ❖ One sliced avocado
- ❖ Four poached eggs
- ❖ Garnish with sesame seeds

❖ Add salt and pepper to taste

GUIDELINES:

1. Put the quinoa and water in a saucepan. After bringing it to a boil, lower the heat, cover, and simmer the quinoa for 15 minutes, or until it is tender.

2. Heat the olive oil in a skillet over medium heat. Add the kale, broccoli, and sweet potato. Sauté the veggies till they get soft.

3. Add salt and pepper to the veggies for seasoning.

4. Divide the cooked quinoa into two bowls to assemble the bowls.

5. Add poached eggs, black beans, avocado slices, and sautéed veggies on top.

6. Add sesame seeds as a garnish for texture.

7. Present the bowls of fertility protein right away.

06. Shrimp and Avocado Bowl

Serves: 2| Prep Time: 15 minutes| Cooking Time: 5 minutes| Total Time: 20 minutes

Nutrition Facts (Per Serving):

500 calories| 30g of protein | 45g of carbohydrates| 20g of fat| 10g of fiber

Ingredients:

- ❖ One pound of peeled and deveined medium
- ❖ Sized shrimp
- ❖ One tablespoon of olive oil

- ❖ One teaspoon each of smoky paprika and garlic powder

- ❖ Add salt and pepper to taste.

- ❖ Cook 1 cup of quinoa.

- ❖ One sliced avocado

- ❖ One cup of chopped cherry tomatoes

- ❖ One diced cucumber

- ❖ 1/4 cup coarsely chopped red onion - 1/4 cup chopped cilantro

- ❖ One lime's juice

- ❖ Hot sauce is optional but adds a kick.

INSTRUCTIONS:

1. Combine the shrimp, garlic powder, olive oil, smoked paprika, salt, and pepper in a bowl.

2. Turn the heat up to medium-high in a skillet. The seasoned shrimp should be cooked for two to three minutes on each side, or until they are opaque and well done.

3. Divide the cooked quinoa into two dishes to form the foundation.

4. Top the quinoa with cooked shrimp, avocado slices, cherry tomatoes, chopped cucumber, red onion, and cilantro.

5. For a cool touch, pour lime juice over the dishes. If you want, add spicy sauce.

6. To blend tastes, gently mix items in each dish.

7. Present the dishes of shrimp and avocado right away.

07. QUINOA AND SWEET POTATO BOWL

Serves: 2| Prep Time: 15 minutes| Cooking Time: 20 minutes| Total Time: 35 minutes

PER-SERVING NUTRITIONAL INFORMATION:

500 calories|- 10g of protein |- 80g of carbohydrates|- 18g of fat| 12g of fiber

INGREDIENTS:

- ❖ 1 cup rinsed quinoa, 2 cups water, 2 medium diced and peeled sweet potatoes, 2 tablespoons olive oil, 1 teaspoon each of cumin and paprika.
- ❖ Half a cup of cherry tomatoes; - Season with salt and pepper.
- ❖ 1/4 cup finely chopped red onion
- ❖ 1/4 cup chopped cilantro
- ❖ 1 sliced avocado
- ❖ One lime's juice
- ❖ Feta cheese garnish, if desired

DIRECTIONS:

1. Put the quinoa and water in a saucepan.

After bringing to a boil, lower the heat, cover, and simmer the quinoa for 15 minutes, or until it is tender.

2. Turn the oven on to 400°F, or 200°C.

3. Combine olive oil, salt, pepper, cumin, and paprika with the diced sweet potatoes. Place them on a baking pan and roast until soft, about 20 minutes.

4. Divide the cooked quinoa into two dishes to form the foundation.

5. Add avocado slices, cherry tomatoes, red onion, cilantro, and roasted sweet potatoes on top.

6. To add a splash of freshness, drizzle lime juice over the dishes.

7. You may optionally top with feta cheese to add more taste.

8. Present the dishes of sweet potatoes and quinoa right away.

08. Salmon and Rice Bowl

Serves: 2| Prep Time: 10 minutes| Cooking Time: 15 minutes| Total Time: 25 minutes

Nutritional Data (per serving):

600 calories| 35g of protein | 55g of carbohydrates| 28g of fat| 6g of fiber

Ingredients:

- ❖ Six ounces each of two salmon fillets
- ❖ Add salt and pepper to taste
- ❖ Combine 1 tablespoon olive oil,
- ❖ 1 cup of cooked brown rice,
- ❖ 1 cup steamed broccoli florets,

- ❖ 1 chopped carrot, and 1/2 sliced cucumber.

- ❖ Two tsp soy sauce

- ❖ One tablespoon each of sesame oil, rice vinegar, and honey

- ❖ One teaspoon of honey

- ❖ Sesame seeds for garnish

- ❖ Chopped green onions for garnish

INSTRUCTIONS:

First, preheat the oven to 400°F, or 200°C.

2. Use salt and pepper to season the salmon filets. Heat the olive oil in a pan over medium-high heat. After searing the salmon for two to three minutes on each side, place it in the oven that has been warmed and bake it for a further ten minutes, or until it is cooked through.

3. Distribute cooked brown rice between two

dishes to create the foundation.

4. Place cucumber slices, julienned carrot, and steam-cooked broccoli on top.

5. Combine the soy sauce, rice vinegar, honey, and sesame oil in a small bowl. Over the bowls, drizzle the sauce.

6. Top the rice and veggies with the cooked salmon fillets.

7. Add chopped green onions and sesame seeds as garnish.

8. Present the rice dishes and fish right away.

09. Bean Burger

Serves: 4| Prep Time: 15 minutes| Cooking Time: 10 minutes| Total Time: 25 minutes

Per-serving Nutritional Information:

300 calories| 12g of protein| 50g of carbohydrates| 6g of fat| 12g of fiber

INGREDIENTS:

- ❖ 1/2 cup breadcrumbs
- ❖ 1 can (15 oz) washed and drained of black beans
- ❖ 1/4 cup finely chopped red onion
- ❖ 1/4 cup finely chopped bell pepper
- ❖ 2 minced garlic cloves
- ❖ One teaspoon each of chili powder and cumin
- ❖ To taste, add salt and pepper. Use one tablespoon of olive oil.
- ❖ Four burger buns made entirely of wheat
- ❖ Adding lettuce, tomatoes, avocados, cheese, and sauces is optional.

INSTRUCTIONS:

1. Using a fork or potato masher, roughly mash the black beans in a large basin until they are nearly smooth.

2. Mix the mashed beans with breadcrumbs, red onion, bell pepper, minced garlic, cumin, chili powder, salt, and pepper. Blend until well blended.

3. Create four equal parts out of the mixture, then form them into burger patties.

4. Heat the olive oil in a pan over medium heat. Cook until a golden crust forms, approximately 4–5 minutes on each side for the bean patties.

Toast the burger buns made from whole wheat.

6. Put the bean burgers together with your preferred toppings on the bread.

7. Present the bean burgers right away.

10. BEET SALAD

Serves: 4| Prep Time: 15 minutes| Cooking Time: 45 minutes (if roasting beets)| Total Time: 1 hour (if roasting beets)

PER-SERVING NUTRITIONAL INFORMATION:

180 calories| 5g of protein| 20g of carbohydrates| 10g of fat| 5g of fiber

INGREDIENTS:

- ❖ 4 medium-sized peeled, chopped, and roasted beets
- ❖ 1/2 cup of crumbled feta cheese
- ❖ 2 cups of mixed salad greens (arugula, spinach, or mixed baby greens)
- ❖ 1/4 cup of chopped and toasted walnuts
- ❖ 1/4 cup of balsamic vinaigrette dressing

❖ One tablespoon of olive oil

❖ To taste, add salt and pepper.

INSTRUCTIONS:

1. Preheat the oven to 400°F (200°C) if you are not using precooked beets. Each beet should be wrapped in foil and roasted for 45 minutes or until soft. After they've cooled, peel and chop them.

2. Combine the chopped roasted beets, toasted walnuts, crumbled feta cheese, and mixed salad greens in a big bowl.

3. Combine the olive oil, salt, pepper, and balsamic vinaigrette dressing in a small bowl.

4. Pour the salad with the dressing and gently toss to coat evenly.

5. You may serve the beet salad on a tray or in separate bowls.

DINNER FOR FERTILITY

01. OYSTER CASSEROLE:

Serves: 4| Prep Time: 15 minutes| Cooking Time: 25 minutes| Total Time: 40 minutes

NUTRITIONAL INFORMATION (PER SERVING):

Calories: ~400| Protein: ~15g| Fat: ~30g| Carbohydrates: ~20g| Fiber: ~1g

INGREDIENTS:

- ❖ Two cups of freshly drained oysters
- ❖ One cup of milk; half a cup of butter; and half a cup of all-purpose flour
- ❖ One cup of thick cream
- ❖ 1/4 teaspoon cayenne pepper

- ❖ 1/2 teaspoon salt; 1/4 teaspoon black pepper; and 1 cup of shredded cheddar cheese
- ❖ Half a cup of breadcrumbs
- ❖ Optional chopped parsley garnish

INSTRUCTIONS:

First, preheat the oven to 375°F, or 190°C.

2. Melt butter in a pot over a medium heat. To make a roux, stir in the flour.

3. Stirring constantly, gradually add the milk and heavy cream until the mixture thickens.

4. Add cayenne, black pepper, and salt for seasoning.

5. toss the drained oysters into the sauce with a gentle toss.

6. Pour the oyster mixture into a casserole dish that has been oiled.

7. Evenly distribute shredded cheddar cheese on top.

8. Combine the breadcrumbs with a small amount of melted butter in a small bowl, then top the cheese with it.

9. Bake for approximately 25 minutes, or until the casserole is bubbling and the top is golden brown, in a preheated oven.

10. Before serving, garnish with chopped parsley if preferred.

02. OYSTER STEW:

Serves: 4| Prep Time: 10 minutes| Cooking Time: 15 minutes|Total Time: 25 minutes

Nutritional Information (per serving):

Calories: ~350| Protein: ~20g| Fat: ~25g| Carbohydrates: ~15g| Fiber: ~1g

Ingredients:

- ❖ 12 freshly shucked oysters
- ❖ 1/2 cup unsalted butter
- ❖ 1 big onion, finely diced
- ❖ 2 minced cloves of garlic
- ❖ Four cups of whole milk
- ❖ 1/4 tsp ground nutmeg
- ❖ Salt and pepper to taste
- ❖ Fresh parsley chopped (optional) as a garnish
- ❖ Serve with oyster crackers

Directions:

1. Melt the butter in a large saucepan over medium heat.

2. Add the minced garlic and chopped onions, and sauté until the onions become transparent.

3. Add the full milk and simmer, being careful not to boil, the mixture.

4. Carefully add the oysters to the saucepan, together with their liquid.

5. Add ground nutmeg, salt, and pepper for seasoning. Mix thoroughly.

6. Make sure the oysters are cooked through but not overdone by simmering the stew for ten to fifteen minutes.

7. Turn off the heat and let it a few minutes to rest.

8. If preferred, garnish with freshly cut parsley.

9. Present heated, with oyster crackers beside it.

03. Beef Stuffed Avocado:

Serves: 2| Prep Time: 15 minutes| Cooking Time:15 minutes| Total Time: 30 minutes

Nutritional Information (per serving):

Calories: ~500| Protein: ~25g| Fat: ~35g| Carbohydrates: ~15g| Fiber: ~8g

Ingredients:

- ❖ 1 pound of beef
- ❖ 2 pitted and halved avocados
- ❖ 1 finely chopped small onion
- ❖ 2 minced garlic cloves
- ❖ One teaspoon each of chili powder and cumin
- ❖ Half a cup of cherry tomatoes
- ❖ Season with salt and pepper.
- ❖ Half a cup of cheddar cheese, shredded

❖ Lime wedges for serving

❖ Optional fresh cilantro garnish

DIRECTIONS:

1. Brown the ground beef in a pan over medium heat. Eliminate extra fat.

2. Add minced garlic and chopped onions to the pan and cook until the onions become tender.

3. Add salt, pepper, cumin, and chili powder to the meat mixture. Mix thoroughly.

4. To make a sturdy foundation, trim a little piece from the bottom of each avocado half.

5. Stuff the meat mixture into the halves of avocados.

6. Add shredded cheddar cheese and cherry tomatoes on top.

7. Bake under broil for 5 to 7 minutes, or until the cheese is bubbling and melted.

8. If preferred, garnish with fresh cilantro.

9. Present with slices of lime on the side.

04. WHITE BEAN CHILI:

Serves: 6| Prep Time: 15 minutes| Cooking Time: 30 minutes| Total Time: 45 minutes

PER-SERVING NUTRITIONAL INFORMATION:

350 calories| Protein: around 30 grams| Fat: about 10g| 35g of carbohydrates| Fiber: around 8 grams

INGREDIENTS:

- ❖ 1 pound of chopped, skinless, boneless chicken breasts

- ❖ 2 tablespoons olive oil; One cup of frozen corn kernels
- ❖ 1 big chopped onion; 3 minced cloves of garlic
- ❖ Two 15-ounce cans of rinsed and drained white beans
- ❖ One 4-ounce can of chopped green chilies
- ❖ One teaspoon each of ground cumin and dried oregano
- ❖ Half a teaspoon each of powdered coriander and cayenne pepper (optional)
- ❖ One lime juice; Four cups chicken broth; Salt and pepper to taste
- ❖ Fresh cilantro chopped for garnish
- ❖ Monterey Jack cheese shredded (optional)

GUIDELINES:

1. Heat the olive oil in a big saucepan over medium heat. Cook the chopped chicken until it

becomes brown.

2. Add the minced garlic and chopped onions, and sauté until the onions become tender.

3. Add the ground cumin, ground coriander, dried oregano, chopped green chilies, white beans, and cayenne pepper (if using).

4. Add the chicken broth, season to taste with pepper and salt, and then simmer.

5. Once the flavors have melded, add the frozen corn kernels and simmer for an additional 15 to 20 minutes.

6. Add lime juice and mix just before serving.

7. If preferred, add shredded Monterey Jack cheese over top and garnish with chopped cilantro.

05. Sweet Potato Gnocchi:

Serves: 4| Prep Time: 30 minutes| Cooking Time: 5 minutes| Total Time: 35 minutes

Per-serving Nutritional Information:

About 300 calories| Protein: around 8 grams| Fat: about 1 gram| 65g of carbohydrates| Fiber: around 8 grams

Ingredients:

- ❖ Bake and mash two medium-sized sweet potatoes (approximately 2 cups)
- ❖ One beaten egg
- ❖ Two cups of all-purpose flour, with more for dusting
- ❖ Add salt to taste
- ❖ One-half teaspoon of optional nutmeg

Instructions:

1. Combine the mashed sweet potatoes, beaten egg, and a dash of salt in a large mixing dish.

2. Add the flour gradually and stir until a dough forms.

3. Using a floured surface, knead the dough until it's smooth.

4. Roll the dough into long, thin ropes by dividing it into smaller sections.

5. To create the gnocchi, cut the ropes into bite-sized pieces.

6. Boil a big kettle of water that has been seasoned.

7. Add the gnocchi to the boiling water in small batches and cook for 2 to 3 minutes, or until they float to the top.

8. Move the cooked gnocchi to a serving plate using a slotted spoon.

06. Pumpkin Curry:

Serves: 4| Prep Time: 15 minutes| Cooking Time: 25 minutes| Total Time: 40 minutes

Per-serving Nutritional Information:

250 calories| 4g of protein| Fat: about 20 grams| 20g of carbohydrates| Fiber: around 3 grams

Ingredients:

- ❖ one can (14 oz) coconut milk
- ❖ Two cups peeled and cubed pumpkin
- ❖ One finely chopped onion
- ❖ Two minced garlic cloves
- ❖ One tablespoon red curry paste
- ❖ One teaspoon curry powder
- ❖ 1 tablespoon of vegetable oil
- ❖ 1 cup of vegetable broth

- ❖ 1 teaspoon each of ground turmeric and coriander
- ❖ Salt and pepper to taste
- ❖ Fresh cilantro for decoration
- ❖ Cooked rice for serving

GUIDELINES:

1. Heat the vegetable oil in a big saucepan over medium heat. Add the minced garlic and chopped onions, and sauté until the onions become transparent.

2. Include the ground coriander, turmeric, and curry powder along with the red curry paste. Mix well to blend.

3. Add the cubed pumpkin to the saucepan and toss to coat with the spice mixture.

4. Add the vegetable broth and coconut milk, stirring to mix. Add pepper and salt for

seasoning.

5. Cook, covered, over medium heat for 20 to 25 minutes, or until the pumpkin is soft.

6. Modify the seasoning as needed.

7. Put the cooked rice on top of the pumpkin curry.

8. Add fresh cilantro as a garnish.

07. PUMPKIN POWER SALAD:

Serves: 4| Prep Time: 15 minutes| Cooking Time: 25 minutes (if roasting pumpkin)| Total Time: 40 minutes

Nutritional data (per serving):

Approximately 250 calories| Protein: around 8 grams| Fat: about 12 grams| 30g of carbohydrates| Fiber: about 6g

Ingredients:

- ❖ Four cups of mixed salad greens, such as kale, spinach, and arugula
- ❖ 1/2 cup rinsed and drained chickpeas
- ❖ 1 cup roasted pumpkin cubes
- ❖ 1/4 cup toasted pepitas, or pumpkin seeds
- ❖ 1/4 cup crumbled feta cheese
- ❖ 1/4 cup of cranberries, dried
- ❖ Two teaspoons of dressing (balsamic vinaigrette).
- ❖ To taste, add salt and pepper.

Guidelines:

1. Set the oven temperature to 400°F (200°C) if you aren't using pre-roasted pumpkin chunks. Roast the pumpkin cubes for 20 to 25 minutes, or until they are soft, after tossing them with olive oil, salt, and pepper.

2. Put the mixed greens, chickpeas, roasted pumpkin cubes, toasted pumpkin seeds, crumbled feta, and dried cranberries in a big salad dish.

3. Cover the salad with a drizzle of balsamic vinaigrette dressing and toss to cover.

4. To taste, add salt and pepper for seasoning.

5. Present right away.

08. BEEF LIVER TACOS:

Serves: 4| Prep Time: 15 minutes| Cooking Time: 15 minutes| Total Time: 30 minutes

Per-serving Nutritional Information:

About 300 calories| Protein: around 25 grams| Fat: about 10g| 25g of carbohydrates| Fiber: around 3 grams

Ingredients:

- ❖ One pound of thinly sliced beef liver
- ❖ One thinly sliced onion
- ❖ Two minced garlic cloves
- ❖ One teaspoon each of ground cumin and chili powder
- ❖ One tablespoon of olive oil
- ❖ Eight little corn or flour tortillas
- ❖ Salt & pepper to taste
- ❖ Add-ons: sour cream, salsa, chopped tomatoes, shredded cheese, and lettuce.

Guidelines:

1. In a pan over medium heat, warm the olive oil.

Add the chopped garlic and onions, and sauté until the onions become tender.

2. Place the thinly sliced beef liver in the pan and cook it until it becomes brown all over.

3. Add salt, pepper, chili powder, and powdered cumin for seasoning. Mix well to cover the liver.

4. Follow the directions on the box to reheat the tortillas in a different pan or microwave.

5. Top the tacos with your preferred toppings and the beef liver mixture.

6. Present right away.

09. CHICKEN LIVER STIR FRY

Serves: 4| Prep Time: 15 minutes| Cooking Time: 15 minutes| Total Time: 30 minutes

NUTRITIONAL INFORMATION (PER

SERVING):

Calories: ~250| Protein: ~20g| Fat: ~10g| Carbohydrates: ~15g| Fiber: ~2g

INGREDIENTS:

- ❖ 1 lb chicken livers, cleaned and halved
- ❖ 1 onion, thinly sliced
- ❖ 2 bell peppers, thinly sliced
- ❖ 2 cloves garlic, minced
- ❖ 1 tablespoon soy sauce
- ❖ 1 tablespoon oyster sauce
- ❖ 1 teaspoon ginger, grated
- ❖ 1 tablespoon vegetable oil
- ❖ Salt and pepper to taste
- ❖ Green onions for garnish (optional)
- ❖ Cooked rice for serving

INSTRUCTIONS:

1. Heat vegetable oil in a wok or large skillet over medium-high heat.

2. Add sliced onions and minced garlic, stir-fry until aromatic.

3. Add chicken livers to the wok, cooking until browned on all sides.

4. Toss in sliced bell peppers and grated ginger, continuing to stir-fry for a few more minutes until the peppers are tender-crisp.

5. In a small bowl, mix soy sauce and oyster sauce. Pour the sauce over the chicken liver mixture.

6. Season with salt and pepper to taste. Stir well to coat.

7. Cook for an additional 3-5 minutes, allowing the flavors to meld.

8. Garnish with chopped green onions if desired.

9. Serve the chicken liver stir fry over cooked rice.

10. Turkey Chili

Serves: 6| Prep Time: 15 minutes| Cooking Time: 30 minutes| Total Time: 45 minutes

Per-serving Nutritional Information:

300 calories| 25 grams of protein| Fat: about 10g| 30 grams of carbohydrates| Fiber: around 8 grams

Ingredients:

- ❖ 1 pound ground turkey
- ❖ Diced onion
- ❖ Minced garlic cloves
- ❖ Diced bell pepper

- ❖ One 14-oz can of chopped tomatoes
- ❖ One can (15 oz) of washed and drained kidney beans
- ❖ One can (15 ounces) of rinsed and drained black beans
- ❖ One cup of tinned, frozen, or fresh corn kernels
- ❖ One cup chicken broth
- ❖ Two tablespoons tomato paste
- ❖ Two teaspoons chili powder
- ❖ One teaspoon each of paprika and cumin
- ❖ To taste, add salt and pepper
- ❖ Use olive oil while cooking

GUIDELINES:

1. Heat the olive oil in a big saucepan over medium heat. When the onions are transparent, add the chopped onions and minced garlic and sauté.

2. Add the ground turkey to the saucepan and cook it until browned, breaking it up with a spoon.

3. Add the chopped bell pepper and simmer, stirring, for a few minutes, until it starts to soften.

4. Include the tomato paste, kidney and black beans, corn, and sliced tomatoes. Blend well.

5. Add the chicken stock and season with salt, pepper, paprika, cumin, and chili powder. Mix everything.

6. Simmer the chili for twenty to twenty-five minutes, stirring now and again.

7. Serve hot, adjusting the spice as needed.

Desserts for Fertility

01. Berry Yogurt Bark

Servings: 8| Prep Time: 10 minutes| Cooking Time: 2 hours (freezing time)|Total Time: 2 hours 10 minutes

Per-serving Nutritional Information:

120 calories| 8g of protein| 15g of carbohydrates| 4g of fat| 2g of fiber| 10g of sugars| 20 milligrams of sodium

Ingredients:

- ❖ Two cups of Greek yogurt
- ❖ 1/4 cup maple syrup or honey
- ❖ One cup of mixed berries (strawberries, blueberries, and raspberries)

❖ One teaspoon of vanilla essence

❖ 1/4 cup of granola

GUIDELINES:

1. In a dish, thoroughly mix the Greek yogurt, vanilla extract, and honey (or maple syrup).

2. Use parchment paper to line a baking sheet.

3. Transfer the yogurt mixture onto the paper, making sure it is uniformly distributed to create a thin coating.

4. Top the yogurt layer with granola and mixed berries.

5. Put the baking sheet in the freezer and leave it there until it solidifies, which should take at least two hours.

6. Break the yogurt bark into pieces when it has

frozen.

7. Present and savor!

02. Sweet Potato Bread

Servings: 12 slices| Prep Time: 15 minutes| Cooking Time: 1 hour| Total Time: 1 hour 15 minutes

Per-serving Nutritional Information:

210 calories| 3g of protein| 30g of carbohydrates| 9g of fat| 2g of fiber| 12g of sugars| 260 mg of sodium

Ingredients:

- ❖ 1/2 cup melted unsalted butter
- ❖ 1/2 cup brown sugar
- ❖ 1 cup cooked and mashed sweet potatoes; 2 big eggs
- ❖ 1 3/4 cups all-purpose flour

- ❖ 1 teaspoon vanilla essence

- ❖ One tsp baking soda

- ❖ One-half tsp baking powder

- ❖ Half a teaspoon each of salt and ground cinnamon

- ❖ 1/4 teaspoon of nutmeg, ground

- ❖ 1/4 cup dairy or plant-based milk

- ❖ 1/2 cup chopped nuts (optional: walnuts or pecans)

GUIDELINES:

1. Set the oven's temperature to 175°C/350°F. Oil and dust a 9 x 5-inch loaf pan.

2. Put the mashed sweet potatoes, eggs, brown sugar, melted butter, and vanilla essence in a big basin. Blend until well blended.

3. Combine the flour, baking powder, baking

soda, salt, cinnamon, and nutmeg in another basin.

4. Alternately add the milk and the dry ingredients to the sweet potato mixture gradually. Blend until barely mixed.

5. Stir in the chopped nuts, if using.

6. Transfer the mixture to the loaf pan that has been ready and level the top.

7. Bake until a toothpick inserted in the middle comes out clean, about 60 minutes.

8. Before slicing, let the bread rest fully on a wire rack after letting it cool in the pan for ten minutes.

03. Banana Pudding:

Servings: 8 | Prep Time: 20 minutes | Cooking Time: 10 minutes | Total Time: 30 minutes (plus chilling time)

Per-serving Nutritional Information:

320 calories | 5g of protein | 54g of carbohydrates | 10g of fat | 2g of fiber | 35g of sugars | 180 mg of sodium

Ingredients:

- ❖ 3 cups whole milk
- ❖ 1/4 cup all-purpose flour
- ❖ 1/4 teaspoon salt
- ❖ 3/4 cup granulated sugar.
- ❖ Beat 3 big egg yolks.

- ❖ One teaspoon vanilla essence

- ❖ Two tablespoons unsalted butter

- ❖ Three sliced ripe bananas

- ❖ One box (approximately twelve ounces) of vanilla wafers

- ❖ Optional whipped cream for topping

DIRECTIONS:

1. Combine sugar, flour, and salt in a medium pot.

2. Add milk gradually while whisking to prevent lumps.

3. Cook over medium heat for 8 to 10 minutes, stirring regularly, or until the mixture thickens.

4. Transfer a small quantity of the heated milk mixture to a separate bowl and gradually whisk in the egg yolks, beating constantly. Next, return the egg mixture to the pot while

continuing to stir continuously.

5. Cook the pudding for a further two minutes, or until it thickens.

6. Turn off the heat and mix in the vanilla essence and butter. Let the pudding come to room temperature.

7. Arrange the pudding, cut bananas, and vanilla wafers in a serving dish or individual cups. Iterate through the levels.

8. To let the flavors combine, place in the refrigerator for at least two hours.

9. If preferred, top with whipped cream before serving.

04. BERRY CHEESECAKE

Servings:12| Prep Time: 30 minutes| Cooking Time:1 hour 15 minutes| Total Time: 8 hours

(including chilling time)

Per-serving Nutritional Information:

There are 480 calories| 8g of protein - 35g of carbohydrates| 35g of fat| 2g of fiber| 25g of sugars# 340 mg of sodium

Ingredients: To make the crust:

- ❖ 1/2 cup of crumbs from graham crackers
- ❖ 1/3 cup of butter, melted
- ❖ Two teaspoons of sugar, granulated

Ingredients for the Filling:

- ❖ Four packages (8 ounces each) of softened cream cheese
- ❖ One cup of sugar, grated
- ❖ Four big eggs
- ❖ One tsp of vanilla extract
- ❖ One cup sour cream

* 1/4 cup all-purpose flour

Ingredients for the Berry Topping:

* 1/4 cup of seedless berry jam

* 2 cups of mixed berries (strawberries, blueberries, and raspberries)

Guidelines:

Crust:

1. Set the oven temperature to 325°F (163°C). In a 9-inch springform pan, grease it.

2. Combine sugar, melted butter, and graham cracker crumbs in a bowl. Fill the prepared pan to the brim with the ingredients.

3. For ten minutes, bake the crust. While you make the filling, let it cool.

Filling:

4. Beat cream cheese and sugar together in a large basin until creamy.

5. Beat well after adding each egg, one at a time.

6. Add flour and vanilla essence, stirring just until incorporated.

7. Add sour cream and fold.

8. Cover the crust in the springform pan with the filling.

Bake

9. Bake until the middle is firm, about 1 hour and 15 minutes.

10. After turning off the oven, let the cheesecake in for an extra 60 minutes.

11. Take it out of the oven, then let it come to room temperature.

BERRY TOPPING:

12. Melt the berry jam in a small pot.

13. Gently combine the melted jam with the mixed berries.

14. Top the cheesecake that has cooled with the berry topping.

15 degrees chill. Before serving, place the cheesecake in the refrigerator for at least six hours or overnight.

05. CHOCOLATE BARK

Servings: 12 | Prep Time: 15 minutes | Cooking Time: 0 minutes | Total Time: 1 hour 15 minutes (including chilling time)

NUTRITIONAL INFORMATION (PER

SERVING):

Calories: 180| Protein: 2g| Carbohydrates: 20g| Fat: 11g| Fiber: 3g| Sugars: 14g| Sodium: 5mg

INGREDIENTS:

- ❖ Chopped 12-oz semi-sweet or dark chocolate
- ❖ 1/2 cup chopped nuts (pistachios, almonds, or whatever combination you choose)
- ❖ 1/4 cup of dried fruit (you may use raisins or cranberries).
- ❖ 1/4 cup of coconut shreds
- ❖ Optional flaky sea salt for sprinkling

GUIDELINES:

1. Spread parchment paper on a baking sheet.

2. Using a double boiler or the microwave, melt the chopped chocolate in a heatproof dish, stirring every 20 seconds to ensure it's smooth.

3. Transfer the melted chocolate to the baking sheet that has been prepared, making sure that the layer is uniform.

4. Evenly scatter shredded coconut, dried fruit, and chopped almonds on top of the chocolate.

5. For a sweet-salty contrast, add flaky sea salt if preferred.

6. Refrigerate the baking sheet for at least an hour, or until the chocolate sets all the way through.

7. Break the chocolate bark into pieces when it has hardened.

06. SWEET PROTEIN BITES:

Servings: 16 bites| Prep Time: 15 minutes| Cooking Time: 0 minutes| Total Time: 1 hour (including chilling time)

Nutritional Information (per serving -1 bite):

Calories: 110| Protein: 5g| Carbohydrates: 11g| Fat: 6g| Fiber: 1g| Sugars: 5g| Sodium: 20mg

Ingredients:

- ❖ 1/2 cup protein powder (vanilla or any other flavor you choose)
- ❖ 1 cup rolled oats
- ❖ 1/2 cup of your preferred nut butter (almond, peanut, etc.)
- ❖ One-third cup of maple syrup or honey
- ❖ One tsp of vanilla extract
- ❖ 1/4 cup chips made with dark chocolate

- ❖ 1/4 cup chopped nuts (almonds, walnuts, or whatever combination you choose).

- ❖ 1/4 cup of shredded coconut without sugar (optional)

GUIDELINES:

1. Combine protein powder and rolled oats in a big bowl.

2. Stir in vanilla extract, nut butter, and honey (or maple syrup). Blend until well blended.

3. Stir in the shredded coconut, chopped almonds, and dark chocolate chips (if using).

4. To make the mixture simpler to handle, chill it for at least 30 minutes after it has been well mixed.

5. Once the dough has cooled, divide it into little sections and shape them into bite-sized balls.

6. Transfer the tasty protein bits to a tray lined

with parchment paper.

7. To make the bites firmer, place them in the refrigerator for a further half hour.

8. Keep refrigerated in an airtight container.

07. PUMPKIN PIE

Servings: 8 slices| Prep Time: 15 minutes| Cooking Time: 45-50 minutes| Total Time: 1 hour 30 minutes (including chilling time)

NUTRITIONAL INFORMATION (PER SERVING -1 SLICE):

Calories: 320| Protein: 6g| Carbohydrates:

38g| Fat: 16g| Fiber: 2g| Sugars: 20g| Sodium: 300mg

INGREDIENTS: PIE CRUST INGREDIENTS:

- ❖ 1/4 cup cold water
- ❖ 1/2 cup chilled and cubed unsalted butter
- ❖ 1 1/4 cups all-purpose flour
- ❖ 1/4 teaspoon salt
- ❖ 1 tablespoon of granulated sugar

FOR THE PUMPKIN FILLING:

- ❖ One fifteen-ounce can of pumpkin puree; two-thirds cup of packed brown sugar; two tablespoons of ground cinnamon
- ❖ 1/2 teaspoon of powdered nutmeg
- ❖ 1 teaspoon of ground ginger
- ❖ 1/4 teaspoon of cloves, ground
- ❖ One-half teaspoon salt—three big eggs
- ❖ One cup of evaporated milk

GUIDELINES:

PIE CRUST:

1. Pulse the flour, salt, and sugar in a food processor. Pulse in the cold butter until the mixture looks like coarse crumbs.

2. Pulse the dough until it comes together, then gradually add the cold water.

3. Form the dough into a disk, cover it with plastic wrap, and chill for a minimum of half an hour.

4. Turn the oven on to 375°F, or 190°C.

5. Using a floured surface, roll out the cold dough and transfer it to a 9-inch pie plate. Cut the edges off.

PUMPKIN FILLING

6. To make the pumpkin filling, combine the

pureed pumpkin, brown sugar, cloves, nutmeg, cinnamon, ginger, and salt in a big bowl.

7. Add the eggs one at a time, thoroughly mixing each one in.

8. Stir in the evaporated milk gradually until smooth.

9. Fill the prepared pie crust with the pumpkin filling.

BAKE:

10. Bake for 45 to 50 minutes, or until the middle is firm, in a preheated oven.

11. Let the pie cool entirely on a cooling rack made of wire.

Cool: 12. Allow to cool for a minimum of two hours before serving.

08. FERTILITY COOKIES

Servings: Approximately 18 cookies| Prep Time: 15 minutes| Cooking Time: 10-12 minutes| Total Time: 27 minutes

NUTRITIONAL DATA (ONE COOKIE PER SERVING):

150 calories| 3g of protein| 14g of carbohydrates| 10g of fat| 2g of fiber| Sugars: 7 grams| 40 milligrams of sodium

INGREDIENTS:

- ❖ 1/4 cup flaxseed meal
- ❖ 1/2 cup almond flour
- ❖ 1 cup rolled oats
- ❖ One-fourth cup of chia seeds
- ❖ 1/2 cup of chopped nuts, either almonds or walnuts
- ❖ One-fourth cup of pumpkin seeds
- ❖ Half a teaspoon of ground cinnamon

- ❖ 1/4 tsp salt

- ❖ 1/2 cup melted coconut oil

- ❖ 1/4 cup maple syrup or honey

- ❖ One big egg, one tsp vanilla essence, and half a cup of dried fruit (apricots, cranberries, or raisins)

GUIDELINES:

1. Set the oven's temperature to 175°C/350°F. Use parchment paper to line a baking sheet.

2. Put rolled oats, flaxseed meal, almond flour, chia seeds, chopped almonds, pumpkin seeds, cinnamon, and salt in a big bowl.

3. Combine the melted coconut oil, egg, vanilla extract, and honey (or maple syrup) in another dish.

4. Combine the wet and dry components, mixing them well.

5. Gently fold the dry fruits into the cookie dough until they are uniformly included.

6. Using a tablespoon-sized scoop, arrange dough parts on the baking sheet that has been prepared, allowing space between each cookie.

7. Using the back of a spoon, gently flatten each cookie.

8. Bake for 10 to 12 minutes, or until the edges are golden brown, in a preheated oven.

9. Let the cookies rest for a few minutes on the baking sheet, then move them to a wire rack to finish cooling.

09. WATERMELON SORBET:

Servings: 6| Prep Time:15 minutes| Cooking

Time: 0 minutes| Total Time: 4 hours 15 minutes (including freezing time)

NUTRITIONAL INFORMATION (PER SERVING):

Calories: 90| Protein: 1g| Carbohydrates: 23g| Fat: 0g | Fiber: 1g| Sugars: 20g| Sodium: 0mg

INGREDIENTS:

- ❖ 1/2 cup granulated sugar
- ❖ 2 tablespoons fresh lime juice
- ❖ 6 cups cubed seedless watermelon
- ❖ Mint leaves as an optional garnish

GUIDELINES:

1. Fill a food processor or blender with the diced watermelon.

2. Blend until liquid and smooth.

3. To get rid of any seeds or pulp, strain the watermelon puree into a basin using a fine-mesh sieve.

4. To make simple syrup, combine the sugar and lime juice in a small saucepan and cook over medium heat until the sugar dissolves.

5. Allow the syrup to reach room temperature.

6. Combine the strained watermelon puree with the simple syrup.

7. Transfer contents to a shallow dish, cover with plastic wrap, and place in the freezer for about two hours.

8. After two hours, stir the liquid and break up any ice crystals with a fork. Continue this process every two to three hours until the sorbet has a smooth, scoopable consistency.

9. Spoon the sorbet into serving plates once it has completely frozen.

10. If wanted, garnish with mint leaves and serve right away.

10. BROWNIES:

Servings: 12 brownies | Prep Time: 15 minutes | Cooking Time: 25-30 minutes | Total Time: 45-50 minutes

NUTRITIONAL INFORMATION (PER SERVING):

Calories: 380 | Protein: 4g | Carbohydrates: 50g | Fat: 20g | Fiber: 2g | Sugars: 35g | Sodium: 130mg

INGREDIENTS:

- ❖ 1 cup melted unsalted butter

- ❖ Two cups of powdered sugar

- ❖ Four big eggs

- ❖ One tsp of vanilla extract

- ❖ One cup of flour (all-purpose)

- ❖ 1/2 cup powdered cocoa

- ❖ One-half tsp baking powder

- ❖ One-half teaspoon of salt

- ❖ One cup of chocolate chips, if desired

- ❖ 1/2 cup chopped nuts (optional: walnuts or pecans)

INSTRUCTIONS:

1. Set the oven's temperature to 350°F (175°C). Coat a 9 x 13-inch baking pan with oil and flour.

2. Combine the sugar and melted butter in a big basin and mix them well.

3. Beat well after each addition of eggs, one at a time.

4. Add the vanilla essence and stir.

5. Combine the flour, baking powder, cocoa powder, and salt in another basin.

6. Mixing until just incorporated, gradually add the dry ingredients to the wet components.

7. You may optionally mix in chopped nuts and chocolate chips.

8. Evenly distribute the batter into the baking pan that has been prepared.

9. Bake for 25 to 30 minutes in a preheated oven, or until a toothpick inserted in the middle emerges with a few moist crumbs attached.

10. Before slicing the brownies into squares, let them cool in the pan.

Snacks for Fertility

01. Granola Bars:

Serves: 12 bars| Prep Time: 15 minutes| Cooking Time: 20 minutes| Total Time: 35 minutes

Nutritional Information (per serving):

Calories: 200| Protein: 5g| Fat: 10g| Carbohydrates: 25g| Fiber: 3g| Sugar: 10g

Ingredients:

- ❖ 1 cup chopped nuts (almonds or walnuts); 2 cups rolled oats
- ❖ Half a cup of maple syrup or honey
- ❖ 1/4 cup of nut butter, such as peanut or almond butter

- ❖ 1/4 cup melted coconut oil

- ❖ Half a teaspoon of cinnamon; One teaspoon of vanilla essence

- ❖ 1/4 teaspoon salt

- ❖ 1/2 cup dried fruits (such as cranberries or raisins) as an optional ingredient

- ❖ 1/4 cup dark chocolate chips are optional.

GUIDELINES:

1. Set the oven's temperature to 175°C/350°F. Place parchment paper into a baking dish.

2. Place chopped nuts and rolled oats in a big bowl.

3. Melt the coconut oil, nut butter, and honey (or maple syrup) in a skillet over low heat. Blend until a smooth consistency is achieved.

4. Take the pot off of the burner and mix in the

salt, cinnamon, and vanilla essence.

5. After adding the liquid mixture to the oats and almonds, whisk everything together well. If desired, add chocolate chips and dried fruits.

6. Pour the mixture onto the baking dish that has been prepared, being sure to push down firmly to form a uniform layer.

7. Bake for 20 minutes, or until the edges are golden brown, in a preheated oven.

8. Let the granola bars cool fully before slicing them into twelve pieces.

02. MACARONI SALAD CRISPS:

Serves: 6 servings| Prep Time: 20 minutes| Cooking Time: 10 minutes| Total Time: 30 minutes

NUTRITIONAL INFORMATION (PER SERVING):

Calories: 350| Protein: 10g| Fat: 20g|
Carbohydrates: 30g| Fiber: 3g| Sugar: 5g

INGREDIENTS:

- ❖ 1 cup mayonnaise
- ❖ 1/4 cup Dijon mustard
- ❖ 1/4 cup apple cider vinegar
- ❖ 1 tablespoon sugar
- ❖ 2 cups cooked and chilled elbow macaroni
- ❖ 1/2 cup diced red bell pepper
- ❖ 1 cup finely chopped celery
- ❖ Salt and pepper to taste
- ❖ 1/2 cup chopped green bell pepper
- ❖ 1/4 cup finely chopped red onion
- ❖ 1/4 cup minced fresh parsley

- ❖ 1 cup shredded cheddar cheese

- ❖ One cup of crumbled crispy bacon

- ❖ Optional: 1/2 cup finely chopped pickles

GUIDELINES:

1. Put cooked macaroni, apple cider vinegar, Dijon mustard, mayonnaise, sugar, salt, and pepper in a big bowl. Blend well.

2. Include chopped parsley, red onion, green and red bell peppers, and celery in the macaroni mixture. Mix well until well blended.

3. Gently stir in the crumbled bacon and cheddar cheese. If you'd like, add chopped pickles.

4. To enable the flavors to mingle, refrigerate the macaroni salad for at least an hour.

5. Turn the oven on to 375°F, or 190°C.

6. Evenly distribute the macaroni salad to form a thin layer on a baking sheet.

7. Bake for ten minutes, or until the edges are crispy and golden brown.

8. Let cool before slicing the macaroni salad crisps into small pieces.

03. Veggies Medley

Serves: 4 | Prep Time: 10 minutes | Cooking Time: 15 minutes | Total Time: 25 minutes

Nutritional Information (per serving):

Calories: 120 | Protein: 3g | Carbohydrates: 15g | Fat: 7g | Fiber: 5g

Ingredients:

- ❖ Two cups of florets of broccoli
- ❖ One cup of baby carrots,

- ❖ One bell pepper,

- ❖ One zucchini,

- ❖ One cup of cherry tomatoes,

- ❖ One bell pepper cut in half

- ❖ Two teaspoons of olive oil

- ❖ Two minced garlic cloves

- ❖ One tsp of dehydrated oregano

- ❖ A single tsp of dried thyme

- ❖ To taste, add salt and pepper.

- ❖ Optional: Parmesan cheese, grated, as a garnish

Guidelines:

1. Heat the olive oil in a big skillet or pan over medium-high heat.

2. Once aromatic, add the minced garlic and sauté it for around 30 seconds.

3. Add sliced bell pepper, zucchini, split baby

carrots, and broccoli florets to the pan. Simmer the veggies for 8 to 10 minutes, stirring now and again, until they are soft but not mushy.

4. Include the cherry tomatoes, salt, pepper, dry thyme, and oregano. Simmer for a further three to five minutes, or until tomatoes begin to soften slightly.

5. Taste and adjust spices.

6. Spoon the vegetable medley onto a platter for serving.

7. For added taste, you may optionally top with grated Parmesan cheese.

8. You can also serve it over cooked rice or quinoa as a side dish.

04. Pumpkin Hummus

Serves: 6 | Prep Time: 10 minutes | Cooking Time: 0 minutes | Total Time: 10 minutes

Nutritional Information (per serving):

Calories: 150 | Protein: 5g | Carbohydrates: 15g | Fat: 9g | Fiber: 4g

Ingredients:

- ❖ 1 can (15 oz) rinsed and drained chickpeas
- ❖ One cup of pureed canned pumpkin
- ❖ One-fourth cup tahini
- ❖ two minced garlic cloves
- ❖ Two tsp olive oil
- ❖ One lemon's juice
- ❖ One teaspoon of cumin powder
- ❖ Half a teaspoon of paprika

❖ To taste, add salt and pepper.

❖ Not required: Garnish with toasted pumpkin seeds

GUIDELINES:

1. Place the chickpeas, pumpkin puree, tahini, minced garlic, olive oil, lemon juice, paprika, ground cumin, and salt and pepper in a food processor.

2. Using a spatula to scrape down the processor's sides as necessary, pulse the mixture until it is smooth and creamy.

3. Use your taste buds to adjust the spices to your liking.

4. You may adjust the consistency of the hummus by adding more olive oil or a small amount of water if it is too thick.

5. Spoon the hummus made from pumpkin onto a

serving dish.

6. For an optional textural boost, top with roasted pumpkin seeds.

7. Accompany with your preferred dipping sauces, pita bread, or vegetable sticks.

05. Quinoa Dinner Side

Serves: 4 | Prep Time: 10 minutes | Cooking Time: 15 minutes | Total Time: 25 minutes

Nutritional Information (per serving):

Calories: 200 | Protein: 6g | Carbohydrates: 30g | Fat: 6g | Fiber: 4g

Ingredients:

- ❖ One cup of washed quinoa

❖ Two cups water or veggie broth

❖ One tablespoon olive oil

❖ One finely sliced onion

❖ Two minced garlic cloves

❖ One sliced bell pepper

❖ One diced zucchini

❖ One teaspoon each of paprika and cumin

❖ Season with salt and pepper - Garnish with fresh parsley

GUIDELINES:

1. Bring water or vegetable broth to a boil in a saucepan. When the quinoa is cooked and the liquid has been absorbed, add it, lower the heat to low, cover it, and simmer for 15 minutes.

2. Heat the olive oil in a big skillet over medium heat. Sauté the chopped onion until it becomes

transparent.

3. Fill the pan with chopped bell pepper, diced zucchini, and minced garlic. Sauté the veggies for a further five minutes, or until they are soft.

4. Add the cooked quinoa, salt, pepper, cumin, and paprika. Simmer for a further two to three minutes to let the flavors combine.

5. Before serving, garnish with fresh parsley.

06. Sunflower Seed Chips

Serves: 4 | Prep Time: 10 minutes | Cooking Time: 20 minutes | Total Time: 30 minutes

Nutritional Information (per serving):

Calories: 180 | Protein: 6g | Carbohydrates: 5g | Fat: 16g | Fiber: 3g

INGREDIENTS:

- ❖ One cup of uncooked sunflower seeds
- ❖ One tablespoon of olive oil
- ❖ one tsp powdered garlic
- ❖ One tsp powdered onion
- ❖ One-half tsp smoked paprika
- ❖ Add salt to taste.

GUIDELINES:

1. Set the oven's temperature to 175°C/350°F.

2. Toss sunflower seeds with olive oil, smoked paprika, onion, garlic, and salt in a bowl until well coated.

3. On a baking sheet covered with parchment paper, arrange the seasoned sunflower seeds in a single layer.

4. Bake, stirring regularly, for 15 to 20 minutes in a preheated oven, or until the sunflower seeds are crispy and golden brown.

5. Take out of the oven and let the chips with sunflower seeds to cool fully before serving.

07. Asparagus Casserole

Serves: 6 | Prep Time: 15 minutes | Cooking Time: 25 minutes | Total Time: 40 minutes

Nutritional Information (per serving):

Calories: 350 | Protein: 20g | Carbohydrates: 15g | Fat: 25g | Fiber: 3g

Ingredients:

- ❖ 1 pound of freshly trimmed and bite-sized asparagus
- ❖ Two cups of cooked, shredded chicken
- ❖ One cup of cooked quinoa
- ❖ One cup of cheddar cheese, shredded
- ❖ one-half cup mayonnaise
- ❖ Half a cup of sour cream
- ❖ 1/4 cup of Parmesan cheese, grated
- ❖ one minced garlic clove
- ❖ One tsp Dijon mustard
- ❖ To taste, add salt and pepper.
- ❖ Half a cup of breadcrumbs, optional for garnish

GUIDELINES:

1. Turn the oven on to 375°F, or 190°C.

2. To halt the cooking process, blanch the asparagus in boiling water for two minutes

before transferring it to an ice bath. After draining, put it away.

3. Combine cooked quinoa, shredded chicken, mayonnaise, sour cream, Parmesan cheese, minced garlic, Dijon mustard, salt, and pepper in a large mixing dish. Blend well.

4. Add the blanched asparagus and fold gently.

5. Spoon the mixture into a casserole dish that has been oiled.

6. For an optional crunchy topping, scatter breadcrumbs on top.

7. Bake the casserole for 25 minutes, or until it's bubbling hot, in a preheated oven.

8. Before serving, let it cool for a few minutes.

08. Chips and Dips Platter

Serves: 4-6 | Prep Time: 15 minutes | Cooking Time: 10 minutes (if making homemade chips) | Total Time: 25 minutes

Nutritional Information (per serving):

Calories: 350 | Protein: 10g | Carbohydrates: 30g | Fat: 22g | Fiber: 5g

Ingredients:

- ❖ 1 cup of corn chips
- ❖ One bag (10 ounces) Six tiny corn tortillas, sliced into wedges, or store-bought tortilla chips
- ❖ Two tsp olive oil
- ❖ One tsp of chili powder
- ❖ Add salt to taste.

REGARDING THE DIPS:

- ❖ 1 Avocado
- ❖ 1/4 cup coarsely chopped red onion
- ❖ 2 ripe avocados
- ❖ one-fourth cup of chopped tomatoes
- ❖ one minced garlic clove
- ❖ one lime's juice
- ❖ To taste, add salt and pepper.

2. SALSA:

- ❖ 1 cup finely chopped tomatoes
- ❖ 1/4 cup of coarsely chopped red onion
- ❖ 1/4 cup freshly chopped fresh cilantro
- ❖ 1 jalapeño with seeds removed
- ❖ one lime's juice
- ❖ Add salt to taste.

3. DIP DE QUESO:

- ❖ One cup of cheddar cheese, shredded

- ❖ Two tablespoons of all-purpose flour and half a cup of milk

- ❖ One tablespoon of butter without salt

- ❖ Half a teaspoon of cumin

- ❖ Half a teaspoon of red pepper flakes

- ❖ To taste, add salt and pepper.

GUIDELINES: REGARDING THE CHIPS:

1. Turn the oven on to 375°F, or 190°C.

2. Toss tortilla wedges with olive oil, chili powder, and salt if you're creating handmade chips. Place them on an oven tray.

3. Bake the chips for 8 to 10 minutes, or until they are crispy and brown.

REGARDING THE DIPS:

1. GUACAMOLE: Mash avocados, chopped tomato, red onion, minced garlic, lime juice, salt, and pepper in a bowl. Blend well.

2. Salsa: Combine chopped tomatoes, red onion, cilantro, jalapeño, lime juice, and salt in another bowl.

3. Queso Dip:

1. Melt butter in a pot over a medium heat. Add flour and whisk until smooth.
2. To prevent lumps, add the milk gradually while whisking constantly.
3. Once the cheese has melted and the mixture is smooth, add the shredded cheddar cheese, cumin, chili powder, salt, and pepper and stir.

Position the Platter:

1. In the middle of a large dish, arrange the tortilla chips.

2. Place bowls of salsa, queso dip, and guacamole around the chips.

3. Present right away and enjoy!

09. Crispy Asparagus

Serves: 4 | Prep Time: 10 minutes | Cooking Time: 15 minutes | Total Time: 25 minutes

Nutritional Information (per serving):

Calories: 120 | Protein: 5g | Carbohydrates: 10g | Fat: 7g | Fiber: 3g

Ingredients:

- ❖ 1 bunch of freshly cut asparagus
- ❖ half a cup of breadcrumbs
- ❖ 1/4 cup of Parmesan cheese, grated
- ❖ Two tsp olive oil
- ❖ one tsp powdered garlic
- ❖ One-half tsp smoked paprika
- ❖ To taste, add salt and pepper.
- ❖ slices of lemon to serve (optional)

Guidelines:

1. Set the oven temperature to 425°F (220°C).

2. Place breadcrumbs, grated Parmesan cheese, smoked paprika, garlic powder, salt, and pepper on a shallow plate.

3. Toss the trimmed asparagus to ensure uniform coating after drizzling it with olive oil.

4. Coat each spear of asparagus with the breadcrumb mixture, pressing the breadcrumbs firmly to stick to the asparagus.

5. Transfer the coated asparagus to a parchment paper-lined baking sheet.

6. Bake the asparagus for 12 to 15 minutes, or until golden brown and crispy, in a preheated oven.

7. Take it out of the oven and give it some time to cool.

8. You may optionally serve the fried asparagus with lemon wedges.

10. Fertility Charcuterie Board

Serves: 6-8 | Prep Time: 20 minutes | Cooking Time: 0 minutes | Total Time: 20 minutes

Nutritional Information (per serving):

Calories: 350 | Protein: 12g | Carbohydrates: 30g | Fat: 20g | Fiber: 5g

Ingredients:

- ❖ 1 cup mixed nuts, including pistachios, walnuts, and almonds.
- ❖ One cup of dried fruits (dates, figs, and apricots)
- ❖ One cup of different cheeses (goat cheese, cheddar, brie)

- ❖ One cup of crackers made with whole grains

- ❖ One cup of fresh fruit (apples, berries, and grapes)

- ❖ half a cup of dark chocolate, split up

- ❖ 1/4 cup of honey

- ❖ 1/4 cup green and black olives

- ❖ One-fourth cup hummus

- ❖ one-fourth cup of Greek yogurt

- ❖ Fresh herbs (like thyme and rosemary) for garnish

GUIDELINES

1. Spread out on a large plate or serving board a selection of nuts, dried fruits, cheeses, crackers, fresh fruits, dark chocolate, olives, hummus, and Greek yogurt.

2. To add a little sweetness to some of the things on the board, drizzle some honey over them.

3. Arrange small bowls or ramekins, such as Greek yogurt and hummus, on the board.

4. Add fresh herbs as a garnish for further visual interest.

5. Put everything in a visually pleasing and balanced order on the board.

6. Present the fertile charcuterie board right away and savor it as a wonderful and nourishing snack.

Drinks for Fertility

01. Citrus Smoothie

Serves: 2| Prep Time: 10 minutes| Cooking Time: 0 minutes| Total Time: 10 minutes

Nutritional Information (per serving):

Calories: 180| Protein: 7g| Carbohydrates: 40g| Fat: 1g| Fiber: 5g

Ingredients:

- ❖ One orange, cut into segments and peeled
- ❖ One sliced and peeled grapefruit
- ❖ One peeled banana
- ❖ Half a cup of Greek yogurt
- ❖ One cup of cubes

- ❖ One tablespoon of honey, if desired for sweetness
- ❖ Mint leaves as an optional garnish

GUIDELINES:

1. Put the orange and grapefruit segments, banana, Greek yogurt, and ice cubes in a blender.

2. Process on high speed until creamy and smooth.

3. If you want the smoothie to be even sweeter, taste it and add honey. Blend once more to integrate.

4. Fill the glasses with the citrus smoothie.

5. For an added touch of freshness, you may optionally garnish with fresh mint leaves.

6. Serve right away and enjoy the deliciously

refreshing citrus flavor!

02. ACAI SMOOTHIE

Serves: 2| Prep Time: 10 minutes| Cooking Time: 0 minutes| Total Time: 10 minutes

NUTRITIONAL INFORMATION (PER SERVING):

Calories: 250| Protein: 5g| Carbohydrates: 40g| Fat: 10g| Fiber: 8g

INGREDIENTS:

- ❖ 2 packs of frozen acai berry puree
- ❖ 1 banana, peeled
- ❖ 1/2 cup mixed berries (strawberries, blueberries, raspberries)

- ❖ 1 cup unsweetened almond milk

- ❖ 1 tablespoon almond butter

- ❖ 1 tablespoon honey (optional for added sweetness)

- ❖ 1/2 cup granola (for topping, optional)

- ❖ Sliced strawberries and banana (for topping, optional)

- ❖ Chia seeds (for topping, optional)

INSTRUCTIONS:

1. Run the frozen acai packs under warm water for a few seconds to slightly soften.

2. In a blender, combine the acai berry puree, banana, mixed berries, almond milk, and almond butter.

3. Blend on high speed until the mixture is

smooth and creamy.

4. Taste the smoothie and add honey if additional sweetness is desired. Blend again to incorporate.

5. Pour the acai smoothie into glasses.

6. Optionally, top with granola, sliced strawberries, banana, and a sprinkle of chia seeds for added texture.

7. Serve immediately and enjoy the refreshing acai goodness!

03. Hot Chocolate

Serves: 2| Prep Time: 5 minutes| Cooking Time: 10 minutes| Total Time: 15 minutes

NUTRITIONAL INFORMATION (PER SERVING):

Calories: 250| Protein: 8g| Carbohydrates: 30g| Fat: 12g| Fiber: 2g

INGREDIENTS:

- two cups of whole milk
- Two tsp of cocoa powder without sugar added
- Two teaspoons of sugar, granulated
- 1/4 cup chopped or semisweet chocolate chips
- Half a teaspoon of extract from vanilla
- A dash of salt
- whipped cream (optional) as a garnish
- Chocolate shavings (optional) as a garnish

Guidelines:

1. Using a small dish, thoroughly mix the sugar and cocoa powder.

2. Bring the whole milk to a simmer in a saucepan over medium heat, being careful not to boil.

3. Add the sugar mixture and cocoa powder, whisking constantly to prevent lumps.

4. Add the chopped or chocolate chips to the pot and stir the chocolate until it melts completely.

5. Stir in a little amount of salt and vanilla essence.

6. Keep heating the hot chocolate until the appropriate temperature is reached.

7. Fill cups with the hot chocolate.

8. You may choose to add chocolate shavings as a garnish and top with whipped cream.

9. Serve right away and enjoy the cozy warmth of the hot chocolate!

04. Citrus Mocktail

Serves: 2| Prep Time: 10 minutes| Total Time: 10 minutes

Nutritional Information (per serving):

Calories: 60| Protein: 1g| Carbohydrates: 16g| Fat: 0g| Fiber: 1g

Ingredients:

- ❖ One juiced orange
- ❖ 1 Juiced grapefruit

- ❖ One squeezed lemon

- ❖ Two tablespoons (modified to taste) of honey or simple syrup

- ❖ One cup of club soda or sparkling water

- ❖ Cubes of ice

- ❖ Optional citrus slice garnish

- ❖ Optional fresh mint leaves as a garnish

GUIDELINES:

1. Squeeze the orange, grapefruit, and lemon juices, as well as any honey or simple syrup, into a pitcher.

2. Make sure the honey or syrup is well dissolved by giving the mixture a good stir.

3. Pour ice cubes into two glasses.

4. Evenly pour the citrus juice mixture into each glass.

5. For a bubbly twist, top each glass with club

soda or sparkling water.

6. Gently mix the ingredients.

7. As an optional finishing touch, add some lemon segments or fresh mint leaves.

8. Present the zesty mocktail right away and enjoy it!

05. PEANUT BUTTER PROTEIN SMOOTHIE

Serves: 2| Prep Time: 5 minutes| Cooking Time: 0 minutes| Total Time: 5 minutes

NUTRITIONAL INFORMATION (PER SERVING):

Calories: 350| Protein: 25g| Carbohydrates: 30g| Fat: 16g| Fiber: 3g

INGREDIENTS:

- ❖ Two teaspoons of peanut butter

- ❖ One peeled banana - One cup of Greek yogurt

- ❖ One cup of whole milk, or any other kind you choose)

- ❖ A single scoop of vanilla protein powder

- ❖ One tablespoon of honey, if desired for sweetness

- ❖ Ice cubes, if desired.

Guidelines:

1. Put peanut butter, banana, Greek yogurt, milk, and protein powder with vanilla in a blender.

2. Process the mixture at a high speed until it's smooth and well-mixed.

3. If you want the smoothie to be even sweeter, taste it and add honey. Blend once more to integrate.

4. You may combine it with ice cubes if you want a smoother consistency.

5. Fill glasses with the peanut butter protein smoothie.

6. Serve right away and enjoy this tasty and protein-rich smoothie!

06. Herbal Fertility Tea

Serves: 2| Prep Time: 5 minutes| Cooking Time: 10 minutes| otal Time: 15 minutes

Nutritional Information (per serving):

Calories: 5| Protein: 0g| Carbohydrates: 1g| Fat: 0g| Fiber: 0g

Ingredients:

❖ 2 tablespoons of blossoming red clover

- ❖ One tsp red raspberry leaf, one tsp nettle leaf

- ❖ One teaspoon of Vitex chaste tree berries

- ❖ Two cups of water

- ❖ For taste, add lemon or honey (optional).

DIRECTIONS:

1. Place two cups of water in a small saucepan and bring to a mild boil.

2. Add chaste tree berries, red clover blooms, nettle leaves, and red raspberry leaves to the boiling water.

3. Lower the heat to a simmer and allow the herbs to cook for ten minutes.

4. Turn off the heat and pour the tea through a strainer into mugs.

5. Give the tea a few minutes to cool.

6. You may optionally add flavor with honey or lemon.

7. Pour the herbal fertility tea and take pleasure in its relaxing effects.

07. Blueberry Ovulation Smoothie

Serves: 2| Prep Time: 5 minutes| Cooking Time: 0 minutes| Total Time: 5 minutes

Nutritional Information (per serving):

Calories: 250| Protein: 8g| Carbohydrates: 30g| Fat: 12g| Fiber: 8g

Ingredients:

- ❖ 1/2 cup Greek yogurt
- ❖ 1 peeled banana

- 1 cup frozen blueberries

- One-third cup of chia seeds

- 1/2 cup unsweetened almond milk

- 1 teaspoon honey (optional for sweetness)

- 1 tablespoon almond butter

- Ice cubes, if desired

- Optional fresh blueberries as a garnish

GUIDELINES:

1. Put the frozen blueberries, banana, almond butter, chia seeds, Greek yogurt, and unsweetened almond milk in a blender.

2. Process the ingredients at a high speed until they become creamy and smooth.

3. If you want the smoothie to be even sweeter, taste it and add honey. Blend once more to integrate.

4. You may combine it with ice cubes if you want a smoother consistency.

5. Fill glasses with the blueberry ovulation smoothie.

6. For an added pop of color, you may optionally top with fresh blueberries.

7. Pour this nutrient-rich smoothie right away and enjoy it!

08. Chocolate Shake

Serves: 2| Prep Time: 5 minutes| Cooking Time: 0 minutes| Total Time: 5 minutes

Nutritional Information (per serving):

Calories: 400| Protein: 8g| Carbohydrates: 50g| Fat: 20g| Fiber: 2g

INGREDIENTS

- ❖ Two cups of chocolate ice cream
- ❖ One cup of whole milk, or any other kind you choose)
- ❖ One teaspoon of vanilla extract
- ❖ Two tablespoons of chocolate syrup
- ❖ Optional whipped cream for topping
- ❖ Chocolate shavings (optional) as a garnish
- ❖ An optional maraschino cherry as a garnish

GUIDELINES:

1. Put the milk, chocolate syrup, vanilla extract, and chocolate ice cream into a blender.

2. Process the mixture at a high speed until it's

smooth and well-mixed.

3. After tasting the shake, add extra milk or chocolate syrup to suit your preference for sweetness or thickness.

4. Fill the glasses with the chocolate shake.

5. For a traditional touch, you may optionally add whipped cream on top and decorate with chocolate shavings or a maraschino cherry.

6. Serve right away and savor the chocolate shake's creamy sweetness.

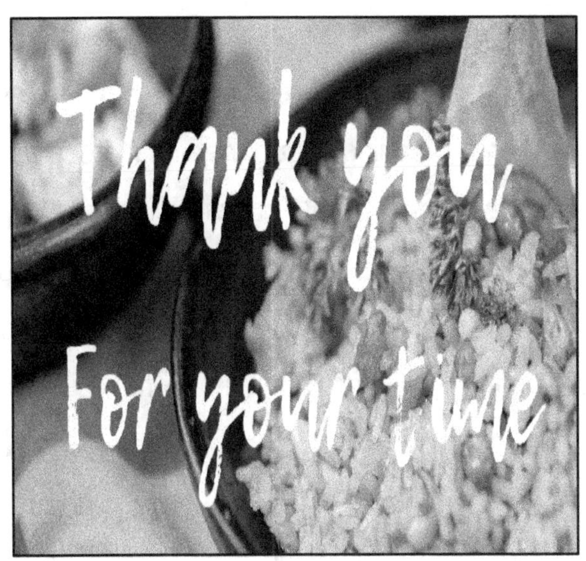

If you're craving swift, health-conscious, and mouthwatering vegetarian meals tailored for the fertility journey of newly married couples, "Fertility Diet Recipes For Newly Married" is your ultimate solution. By embracing these recipes, you gain the key to crafting culinary delights specifically designed to support your fertility goals. Feel empowered to adjust ingredients, adding your personal touch to every dish. Soon, you'll not only have fertility-boosting recipes but also cherished favorites for your private indulgence. This cookbook opens up a world of possibilities, ensuring you meet your dietary goals for fertility without compromising on flavor. Relish the journey to a healthier, more flavorful lifestyle crafted for newlyweds on their fertility path!

Bonus : Grocery Shopping List

Week of: _____________________ Date_____________________________

Recipes to try

Appetizer

Condiments and sauce

Dairy and eggs

Bakery and snacks

Meat and protein

Grains and staples

Canned and packaged goods

Miscellaneous

Notes:

Remember to check pantry for existing items.

Consider any dietary preferences or restrictions

Double-check the recipes for any specific brands or variations.

Week of: _____________________ Date_______________________________

Recipes to try

Appetizer

Condiments and sauce

Dairy and eggs

Bakery and snacks

Meat and protein

Grains and staples

Canned and packaged goods

Miscellaneous